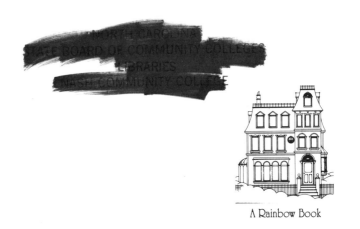

A Rainbow Book

D1526352

Heart Friendly Exercises

Live Longer — Feel Younger

Jack Wexler, M.D.

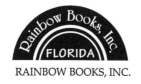

RAINBOW BOOKS, INC.

Library of Congress Cataloging-In-Publication Data

Wexler, Jack, 1913-
    Heart friendly exercises : live longer, feel younger / Jack Wexler.
        p.   cm.
    ISBN 1-56825-049-5
    1. Coronary heart disease — Exercise therapy. I. Title.

RC685.C6 W45 1999
616.1'23062—dc21   99-49138

Heart Friendly Exercises
Live Longer — Feel Younger
by Jack Wexler, M.D.

ISBN 1-56825-049-5 / softcover / $13.00

Publishing industry inquiries (reviewers, retailers, libraries, wholesalers, distributors/media) should be addressed to:

Rainbow Books, Inc.
P.O. Box 430, Highland City, FL 33846-0430
Editorial Offices—
Telephone: (888) 613-BOOK; Fax: (863) 648-4420
Email: RBIbooks@aol.com

Individuals' Orders: (800) 356-9315; Fax: (800) 242-0036; Online: (http://www.) upperaccess.com, amazon.com, barnesandnoble.com

Printed in the United States of America.

DEDICATION

This book is dedicated to my teachers. My college teachers taught me basic science and to understand the complexities of the chemistry of the human body and the world we live in. In medical school, my pre-clinical teachers taught me about the exquisitely organized physiology of the healthy human body. Dr. Frank Apperly who came all the way from Australia taught me how the pathology of disease disrupts the exquisite balance of normal human physiology. My clinical instructors showed me how to attempt to correct the pathology and return the body to a state of health. Finally, my post-graduate mentors, the Nobel Laureates Dr. George R. Minot and Dr. William B. Castle taught me how to apply what I had learned at the bedside for the benefit of the patient. My mentors in Cardiology, Dr. Paul White, Dr. Larry Ellis, Dr. Burton Hamilton and others directed my final career to the study and practice of Cardiology and my interest in the circulation. All of the above have played a part in the development of the heart friendly exercises. I hope they all approve of my project.

CONTENTS

INTRODUCTION

Primitive man did not have the word "exercise" in his vocabulary. However, he unknowingly engaged in vigorous exercise in the pursuit of his prey. When successful, he did not have a vehicle to drive back to his cave. He carried or dragged the prize home. Work and exercise were one and the same. His diet was sparse and lean. In spite of a "healthy diet" and a vigorous lifestyle, he died at an early age from trauma or infection. He did not live long enough to develop coronary artery disease.

It was only about 3,000 years ago that the Greeks distinguished between work for gain or profit and introduced exercise for recreation and fun. They introduced competitive sports that led to the first Olympic games in 776 BC. These games were intended primarily for amusement but consisted of activities that meet current exercise criteria. They not only produced physical fitness but also enhanced the strength and beauty of the human body. People engaged in these activities for about 2,500 years before they knew anything about the circulation of blood in human beings.

In 1616 a British physician described the flow of blood from the heart into the arteries and thence into the veins. Finally, in 1661 an Italian physician described the capillaries through which the blood must pass enroute to the veins leading back to the heart. This completed the journey the blood makes.

In 1768, approximately 150 years after learning about the circulation of the blood, the medical profession became aware that impaired circulation through the coronary arteries was related to the chest pains known as "Angina Pectoris." In time it was observed that vigorous exercise was accompanied by an increase in the speed and volume per minute flow of blood. Some time thereafter it was suggested that this increased blood flow should be helpful to patients with impaired blood flow through the coronary arteries. In recent years clinical observations support the view that exercise may delay the onset of and possibly favorably influence the course of coronary heart disease.

The theory that exercise could increase blood flow to the heart suggested that it could also increase blood flow to the brain. An opportunity to test this assumption occurred when patients, who complained of feeling light headed and unsteady upon getting out of bed in the morning, were relieved of their symptoms by performing a brief series of exercises before getting out of bed. The success of this treatment assumed that the exercises improved the circulation to the brain. The brain was a passive beneficiary of the general increase in the blood flow that resulted from the exercise. The brain did no extra work to gain from the increase in blood flow.

This is not the case with the heart. The heart must participate in the increased work necessary to provide the increase in blood supply that exercising muscles demand. This raises the question whether the benefits to the heart of traditional exercise outweigh the demands placed on the heart by vigorous exercise.

The exercises that are traditionally recommended for prevention or treatment of coronary heart disease are similar to many that were devised by the ancient Greeks. These exercises were devised with no thought of their affect on the circulation or on coronary heart disease, which were unknown at that time. What may have been good for the young Greeks and may be good for most young Americans may not be good for people who have blood vessels narrowed by disease supplying blood to the heart or to the brain.

Exercises that require holding one's breath and straining are generally not part of a usual physical fitness program except for those individuals whose aim is to develop large muscles for professional reasons. These exercises include the once popular isometric exercises and are especially dangerous for patients with impaired coronary circulation. They should not be included in any program intended to benefit the heart or circulation. Even vigorous, generally accepted aerobic exercises should not be haphazardly prescribed for patients with known or suspected disease of the coronary arteries. This risk is unnecessary, especially since recent evidence indicates that the benefits of relatively gentle exercise approach the benefits of vigorous exercise.

The medical profession has now been studying the circulation, coronary heart disease and exercise for over 200 years. It is time to re-examine the relationship between the three in the light of current knowledge. We now realize that the circulation is "the stream of life". When the circulation stops, life stops. The heart is the key player in maintaining the circulation. Exercise is an auxiliary player in maintaining a healthy circulation.

The proper function of the lungs, an essential component of the circulation, is not sufficiently stressed in most physical fitness programs. The lungs help purify the blood and supply the oxygen essential to life. The Heart Friendly

Exercises take advantage of the advances in our understanding of the physiology and anatomy of the heart and blood vessels. Voluntary control of breathing is used to enhance the beneficial effects of exercise on the circulation to the heart and brain.

The following principles characterize this approach:

1. If breathing is placed under voluntary control, it will enhance the benefit of exercise.

2. The circulation can be improved without resorting to vigorous exercises that may be unsafe.

3. It is more cost-efficient for the heart when a large number of muscles are used in relatively mild exercise than when a few muscles are involved in vigorous exercise.

Heart friendly exercises differ from traditional exercise and are especially designed to favor the circulation of blood to the heart and brain. Nonetheless they produce a remarkable increase in muscle tone and strength without excessive exertion. They are appropriate for people of all ages if the intensity of performance is adjusted to the physical condition of each individual upon undertaking the program.

CHAPTER 1

*Exercise,
the Heart Muscle
and the
Skeletal Muscles*

All exercises that consist of repetitive movements of a group of muscles cause an increase in oxygen consumption and are called aerobic exercises. The increased work performed by exercising muscles causes an accumulation of waste products of muscle metabolism and a decrease in the oxygen level in the blood within the muscles. When these waste products and the blood with the decreased oxygen level reach certain receptors in the heart and lungs, they reflexly increase the heart rate, the volume of blood pumped per unit of time and the frequency and depth of breathing. The heart works harder to supply the larger amount of blood needed to provide the increased amount of oxygen and nutrients used up by the muscles in each exercise.

Common aerobic exercises include walking, running, cycling, swimming, various sports and studio aerobics. Each results in increased oxygen consumption and creates the demand for more blood flow to the exercising muscles. Most of the increased blood flow goes to meet the increased needs of the muscles involved in the exercise. This is accomplished by a clever automatic system which shunts blood away from organ systems not "in use" during exercise. For example, the blood flow to the digestive tract is not increased and may even be decreased because we generally do not eat nor digest large amounts of food during exercise. It is wise to avoid exercise after eating except a gentle stroll.

When the heart speeds up, it does so by shortening the rest period between contractions of the heart muscle. During the resting period the heart muscle is "soft" and relaxed and the resistance to blood flow through the coronary arteries to the muscle is at its lowest. *Most of the blood flow to the heart muscle occurs at this time.*

In traditional exercise programs it is recommended that exercise be continued until the heart rate accelerates to a predetermined rate, the "target rate." The target rate is determined by subtracting the person's age from a preset number, 220 beats per minute. The target rate, therefore, gets lower for older people. This is a fortuitous provision to ameliorate untoward affects of decreased blood flow through narrower, older coronary arteries.

The gain in blood flow to the heart muscle when measured against the added work during rapid heart rates may not be cost-effective for the heart. This is of minor significance if the coronary arteries are normal and widely open because the increased blood flow to the heart muscle is still sufficient to compensate for the increased workload on the heart. With narrowed coronary arteries the decrease in resting time may result in inadequate blood supply needed for the heart muscle to meet the increased demand of exercise. The imbalance between increased workload without matching increase in blood supply may prove critical.

Sudden death during exercise can occur if the blood

supply to the heart muscle is inadequate to meet the demands of the moment. Such unfortunate events have been reported even during exercise stress tests conducted under careful monitoring in a cardiac laboratory. The risk of sudden death is increased when the individuals push to attain the target pulse rate.

It is difficult to assess the frequency of such deaths during exercise because many are not reported. However, numerous reports of sudden death during exercise have been reported in the medical literature. Dr. Thompson of the Pittsburgh Heart Institute estimates that six middle aged men per hundred thousand die suddenly during exercise each year. This figure is probably too low because it does not allow for those occurrences that go unreported and excludes women who are not immune to sudden death during exercise.

A group from a hospital in the Netherlands reported in American Journal of Cardiology the successful resuscitation of 17 cardiac arrests (sudden deaths). Ten occurred during sporting events and seven during or just after cardiac stress tests. Fortunately all but two of the 17 cardiac arrests occurred in a hospital setting and were successfully resuscitated. Only two of the 17 were women. The two who were successfully resuscitated away from the hospital were either very lucky or accompanied by a companion who was trained in cardiac resuscitation. The 10 cases that occurred during sporting events were all in the middle to late forties in age. The seven stress test patients were older. In all patients the underlying cause was found to be either known or unsuspected disease of the coronary arteries. In this population sudden death is more likely to occur during vigorous or unaccustomed exercise.

In young people the occurrence of sudden death during

an athletic event is generally due to a congenital cardiac abnormality.

The conclusion expressed by most authors is that the risk of sudden death is low and the benefits of exercise justify the risk. It is doubtful if any of those who had cardiac arrest in settings where resuscitation was not possible or even any of those who were successfully resuscitated would share this conclusion. The heart friendly exercises provide the benefits without the risks of exercise.

In view of the above findings, it would make more sense to adjust the "target heart rate" to the condition of a person's coronary arteries rather than to age of the person. Unfortunately, it is impossible for everyone to know the precise condition of his or her coronary arteries. The heart friendly exercises, therefore, do not use a target heart rate as an endpoint to judge the adequacy of exercise. Any exercise that produces unusual pain in any part of the body should be stopped and the cause for the pain investigated. This does not include normal muscle stiffness and soreness that decreases during the course of the exercises. The non-exhausting heart friendly exercises reduce what little risk of sudden death exists during exercise by avoiding the conditions that are likely to place an unfair load on the heart.

By reducing fear of sudden death, many more who have recovered from a heart attack would continue on exercise programs. Hopefully, some of the 50 percent of Americans who do not engage in any type of exercise may be encouraged to partake in the heart friendly exercises because they are non-exhausting and conveniently performed in the privacy of the bedroom.

It is important to know how the effect of exercise on the heart muscle differs from that on skeletal muscles.

When skeletal muscles contract, as they do during any

exercise, they squeeze the blood out of the smaller veins in the muscles into larger veins that have valves that permit blood to flow only toward the heart. The next muscle contraction forces this blood a little further along its course to the heart.

In this respect the skeletal muscles during exercise act as auxiliary pumps helping the heart. The significance of this auxiliary pump is demonstrated in the following example.

The young cadet, who has been kept too long at rigid attention on the parade ground, may keel over and fall to the ground. The skeletal muscles have not been "pumping" and the blood is pooled in the lower extremities. The heart alone is unable to push sufficient blood against gravity to the brain. Once on the ground, in the horizontal position, blood readily reaches the brain and the embarrassed young man is able to get to his feet.

The simple act of rising onto the toes and contracting the buttocks, as is done in most of the heart friendly exercises, compresses the veins in these large muscles and "squeezes" the blood out of the veins into larger veins enroute to the heart. The brief, non-exhausting contraction of a large muscle mass produces a similar effect that vigorous contraction of a regional group of muscles does without placing a great burden on the heart.

In the heart friendly exercises the effect of the muscle contractions is further enhanced by synchronizing the contraction with inhalation. The rationale for this effect will be easily understood after reading the next chapter. The unique quality of the heart friendly exercises is that they send more blood to the coronary arteries with less physical exertion and therefore less work for the heart. The cost-effective increase in coronary artery blood flow is the most important benefit that exercise offers the heart. Exercise has different benefits for skeletal muscles. Skeletal muscles grow larger, stronger and more efficient as a result of work or repeated exercise. In this and other important respects, the heart muscle is quite different from the skeletal muscles used in work and exercise. The heart muscle works constantly for a lifetime and, in the absence of disease, the heart does not enlarge. If a normal heart enlarged as a result of work, it would soon become too large for the chest cavity with disastrous results.

In most exercise programs the heart works harder primarily to provide the oxygen and nutrients demanded by the exercising skeletal muscles. The increased blood flow also carries off the increased products of muscle metabolism and makes it possible for the muscles to grow bigger and stronger. In the heart friendly exercises, we attempt to make the skeletal muscles work for the heart and only secondarily for their own benefit.

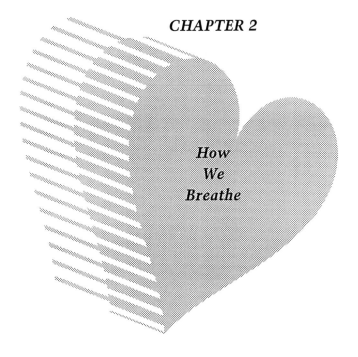

CHAPTER 2

How
We
Breathe

The increase in blood flow to the heart, to exercising muscles or any organ would be of little use if it did not bring with it blood with a fresh supply of oxygen and free of excess carbon dioxide. Healthy lungs are essential for the circulatory system to fulfill its mission. The blood that returns from the exercising muscles to the lungs has an increased amount of carbon dioxide and a decreased amount of oxygen. The high carbon dioxide automatically stimulates the depth and frequency of breathing. The excess carbon dioxide is thus blown off and a fresh supply of oxygen is brought into the lungs more quickly. At the same time other reflexes increase the heart rate which increases the total amount of blood pumped by the heart per minute. The replenished blood enters the heart from the lungs and is carried to the exercising muscles and to other parts of the body. A disproportionate amount of the increased blood flow goes to the exercising muscles to remove the waste products and supply the increase in oxygen demand by the exercising muscles. Normally this takes place without any conscious effort.

It is possible to by-pass this complex process by placing breathing under voluntary control. This makes it possible to determine when and how deeply to breathe without waiting for vigorous muscle action to build up waste products of muscle metabolism that set off the above events.

To accomplish this, we must understand how we breathe. When we breathe in, the muscles of the chest wall contract, causing the ribs to flare out. At the same time the diaphragm contracts and pulls down into the abdominal cavity. This enlarges the chest cavity and creates a negative pressure (a partial vacuum) inside the chest. At this point air with a new supply of oxygen is sucked into the lungs to overcome the partial vacuum. When we let our breath out (exhale, expire) the chest muscles and diaphragm relax. The diaphragm rises into the chest and together with the weight of the chest wall (ribs and muscles) compress the expanded lungs to force out the stale air. Under natural conditions this entire cycle of events takes place automatically.

If we take control of respiration we can coordinate each inspiration with each muscle contraction. The blood flow from the exercising muscles will then reach the chest when there is a partial vacuum in the chest cavity and less resistance to the inflow of blood. Under these conditions, more blood can enter the chest per unit of time than would be possible if the blood arrived during expiration when there is a relatively high pressure within the chest cavity to overcome. This reduces the work the heart must do in pumping the blood along its course to the heart > lungs > heart > coronary arteries. The coordination between inspiration and muscle contraction is possible only in the heart friendly exercises.

The heart friendly program is designed to involve many muscles simultaneously in moderate to light exercises. This avoids involvement of a special group of muscles in vigorous exercise with resultant build up of the waste products that will set off the reflexes described above.

Since the muscles do not work as hard in this voluntary arrangement there will be no physiological reason to divert a large amount of blood to them. As a result relatively more of the increased blood flow is available to the heart and other vital organs. The heart does not work as hard to gain the benefits of the increase in blood flow.

The heart rate need not increase to a target rate. The benefits of an increase in the blood flow are available at a slower heart rate. This means not only less work, but more importantly, less risk for the heart. These differences may not be significant if the coronary arteries are normal, but may be critical if the coronary arteries are narrowed by disease. Most men in their forties and most post-menopausal women have some degree of coronary artery disease.

The heart friendly exercises by-pass the natural reflexes by taking control of the breathing mechanism. In this respect they are an improvement on nature. For those who object to fooling with nature, we point out that if we did not "fool with nature" we would still be living in caves and dying of plague!

Despite their low intensity, the heart friendly exercises increase the size and strength of the skeletal muscles. Most significantly, they extend body flexibility and youthful body movement into the senior years.

The heart friendly exercises avoid the complexity and expense of most programs for physical fitness. They require no special equipment, require only about twenty minutes and are not exhausting. They start while still in bed and are completed in the privacy of the bedroom before other daily duties can interfere with the program. Only approximately half of the American adults engage in any physical fitness program. The heart friendly program may be more suited to the abilities and lifestyle of the average individual than traditional exercise programs.

CHAPTER 3

The Different Types of Exercises

Generally speaking, there are three major types of exercise. All can be performed without the use of any type of equipment. Traditionally these exercises are combined in various proportions in fitness programs to produce the desired result. The weight lifter whose aim is to build huge muscles pursues a program that is quite different from one that the marathon runner would pursue. The exercises are greatly modified and are combined with controlled breathing to create the heart friendly program.

Stretching exercises:

Stretching exercises are aerobic and are generally used as a warm-up for more vigorous aerobic exercises such as jogging. In the heart friendly exercises they are different, more vigorous, and aim to maintain flexibility of the muscles and joints. In this group of the heart friendly exercises, we not only carefully correlate breathing within prescribed movements, we also exercise the muscles used in breathing. Expirations are forced, quick and accompanied by loud grunts or other vocal sounds. If properly executed, they will extend the suppleness of the young body into the senior years.

The Resistance exercises:

These exercises primarily increase muscle strength and mass. They are exemplified by weight lifting, body building machines and the once popular *isometric* exercises.

In *isometrics* the contraction of one muscle group is used to resist the effect of the contraction of an opposing group of muscles. This essentially abolishes any significant movement. Despite the fact that no significant movement results, the muscles are contracting as they do when trying to lift a heavy weight or when pushing against an immovable object.

In *isometric* exercises and all other resistance exercises it is customary to take a deep breath, hold it and strain during the period of exertion. This is a serious disadvantage from a cardiac point of view. The heart is asked to do extra work while fresh blood and oxygen supply to the heart is temporarily decreased because breathing is stopped and the pressure in the chest cavity is greatly increased during the exertion. This is the very time the heart muscle needs more blood and oxygen. Weightlifting machines share this disadvantage. These exercises are not aerobic and are generally excluded in programs intended for heart patients.

The heart friendly exercises convert the isometric exercises to acceptable aerobic status by coordinating the muscle contraction *with inspiration*, when we breathe-in, and fresh oxygen-rich air enters the chest. At the same time, the blood flow reaches the chest while the pressure in the chest cavity is low and proceeds more easily enroute to heart. This procedure converts *isometrics* to a new aerobic form of exercise that we call ***isorobics*** during which an adequate supply of oxygen rich blood reaches the heart. These modified, now aerobic, resistance exercises are used in the heart friendly program to replace weight lifting or special machines. This friendly program produces a remarkable degree of physical fitness for the effort and time expended. No special equipment is required. The exercises may be performed in a matter of 15 to 20 minutes in the privacy of one's bedroom.

The heart friendly exercises may be executed with varying degrees of intensity and should be adjusted to the physical capabilities of the individual. There is no target heart rate. The intensity is increased gradually as tolerated. The appearance of excessive shortness of breath, pain or tightness in the chest is a signal to stop and to decrease the intensity in future sessions. If *any* chest discomfort recurs at the lower intensity, consult your physician.

CHAPTER 4

Heart
Friendly
Exercises

Any exercise may prove difficult to perform at first try but generally will become easier with each attempt. If an exercise causes pain, it should be discontinued unless approved after consultation with a physician. Stiffness and slight soreness is normal after exercise and should diminish with time.

Each exercise is numbered to correspond to the illustration. Read the description and study the illustration before attempting the exercise.

When one exercise is mastered, go to the next one.

Proceed at your own pace until you have mastered all the exercises. Exert sufficient effort with each exercise to produce slight shortness of breath.

After attending to nature's call, return to bed, roll the bed covers down over your legs and you are ready to start your exercise program. When you are familiar with each exercise, aim to complete the entire program without stopping.

THE IN-BED EXERCISES

Exercise 1

Exercise number one will limber up the fingers, wrists and shoulders. The contraction of the muscles in the buttocks and arms helps propel the blood toward the heart and thence to the brain and other organs.

Lie flat on your back, raise the hands and reach for the ceiling with fingers extended. With the mouth open and breathing quietly, alternately make a fist and then briskly extend your fingers. Each time a fist is made, tighten the buttocks and inhale gently. Hold this position for only a moment then extend the fingers and relax the buttocks as you exhale quietly. Breathing should be shallow during this exercise in order to avoid over-breathing and a light-headed feeling.

Repeat this exercise 10 times.

Exercise 1

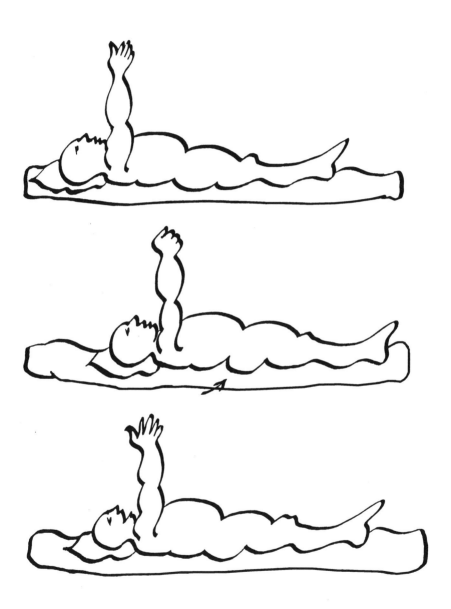

THE IN-BED EXERCISES

Exercise 2

Exercise number two will add to the benefits of exercise number one by promoting and maintaining the flexibility of the wrists.

Without changing position in bed, again raise your arms with fingers extended. This time as fists are made flex the wrists vigorously and tighten the buttocks. Here again all muscle contractions must be timed to coincide with a shallow inhalation.

Repeat this exercise 10 times.

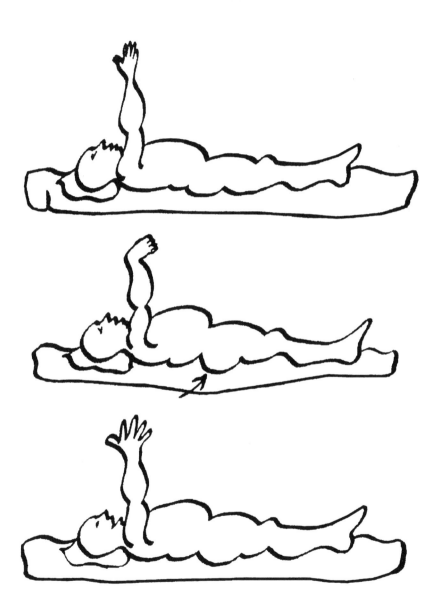

Exercise 2

THE IN-BED EXERCISES

Exercise 3
This exercise adds the involvement of the shoulder joints to the joints of the fingers and wrists.

We start again while lying flat on our back with arms raised and fingers extended, but this time as we make a fist, tighten the buttocks and inhale gently, we rotate the arms inward so that the thumbs move toward each other. We then relax the muscles, exhale gently and return to the starting position.

Repeat this exercise 10 times.

Exercise 3

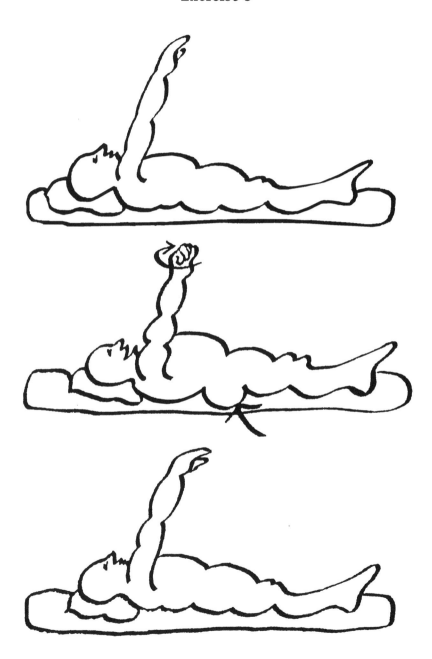

THE IN-BED EXERCISES

Exercise 4

Start as in number three, but this time as we
inhale, make a fist and tighten the buttocks and
rotate the arms outward so that the thumbs move
away from each other. We then relax the muscles,
exhale gently, and rotate the arms inward with
thumbs turning toward each other as we return
to the starting position.

This exercise should be performed 10 times.

*These exercises should get rid of or at least decrease stiff-
ness of the fingers, wrists and shoulders. The fingers will
feel thinner and suppler after these exercises. The tighten-
ing of the buttocks in these and subsequent exercises is
good for the back and will combat the tendency for buttocks to sag as we grow older. At the same time the contraction of these larger muscles squeezes blood from the
muscles toward the heart. These exercises will maintain
flexibility of the fingers, wrists and shoulders.*

Exercise 4

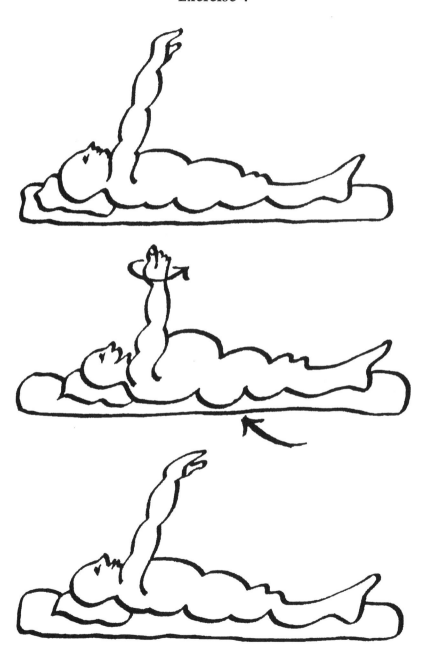

THE IN-BED EXERCISES

Exercise 5

This exercise will stretch the back and muscles in the back of the thighs.

While still in bed, with the bed covers below the knees, keep the legs together and extended. Raise the arms with fingers reaching for the ceiling and *inhale* deeply. Now *exhale* forcefully and simultaneously sit up and grab the toes. The head should be tucked between the arms while reaching for the toes. Return slowly onto the back, as you again raise your arms and inhale. Exhale forcibly and noisily through pursed lips and again reach for the toes. If you can not reach to your toes despite the forced expiration, go as far as you can. The muscles will loosen up after several efforts and permit you to reach the toes.

Repeat this exercise at least five times.

Exercise 5

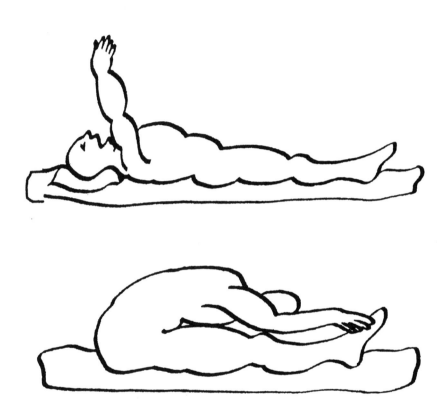

THE IN-BED EXERCISES

Exercise 6

In this exercise a continuous "circle" of the body is formed as the hands grasp and hold firmly to the feet. The powerful leg muscles extend the ankles and push the toes forward producing tension and stretching in the entire "circle." The additional short expiratory efforts empty the base of the lungs and replace stale air with fresh oxygen-bearing air. You will be able to take a deeper breath as you recline after these additional, forced expirations. Similar clearing of stale air is attained in traditional exercise only after vigorous exercise produces hyperventilation. The effort necessary to produce this degree of hyperventilation by standard aerobic exercises is beyond the ability of many and dangerous for those with impaired coronary artery circulation.

Start as in exercise number five, but this time as you exhale forcefully and simultaneously, sit up, grasp the feet and pull briefly on the feet as the powerful leg muscles push the feet away. After blowing "all" your breath out, add three or more short, forced expiratory efforts coordinated with each extension of the ankles to force a little more stale air out of the lungs. Feel the pull and stretching of the thigh and back muscles during this exercise. Return slowly onto the back, as you again raise your arms and inhale.

Repeat this exercise at least five times.

Exercise 6

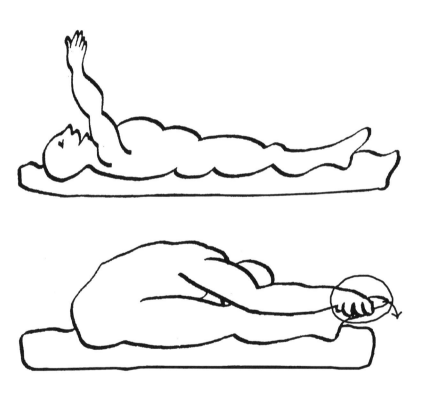

THE IN-BED EXERCISES

Exercise 7

This exercise will tighten the abdominal muscles and strengthen the back muscles, but may be contraindicated if you have a back problem. Consult your physician if this exercises causes back pain.

With arms extended and fingers pointing to the ceiling, take a deep breath. Exhale forcefully as the legs are raised with knees stiff until the toes touch the palms of the hands. Then inhale slowly, make a fist and _slowly_ lower the legs. Stop just before the feet touch the bed.

Repeat this exercise five times.

Exercise 7

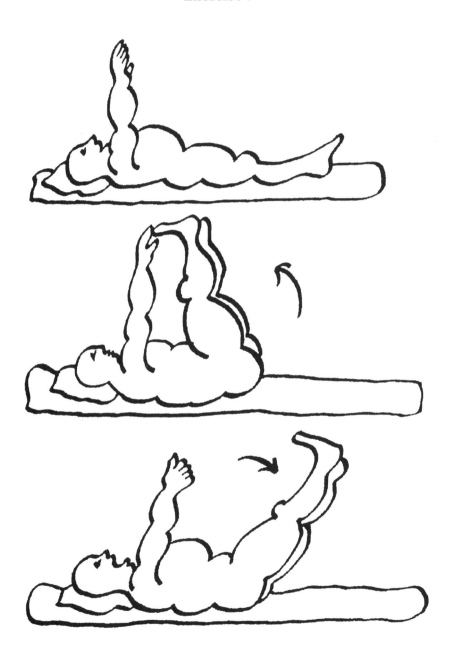

THE IN-BED EXERCISES

Exercise 8
This exercise will enhance flexibility of the hip joints.

With arms extended and fingers pointing to the ceiling, take a deep breath. Exhale while raising first the right leg and try to kick the left palm, then *slowly* lower the leg while inhaling. Repeat with the left foot kicking the right palm.

After a few sessions, the above exercises can be completed in a few minutes. You then feel ready to get out of bed and in the mood to continue with the remainder of the heart friendly exercises. You should be aware that you have coordinated muscle contractions with inspiration. This will become more obvious in all of the remaining heart friendly exercises.

Exercise 8

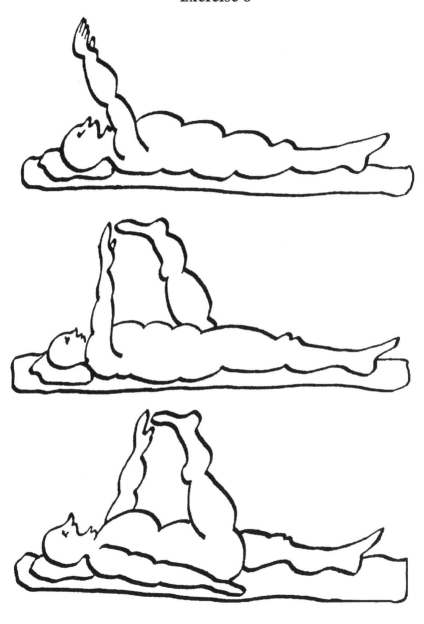

CHAPTER 5

The Stretching and Flexing Exercises

People limited in the degree of flexibility may find some of the exercises difficult at the start. Persevere and you will improve with time. Do not force yourself to the point of pain.

If after a week or two you notice no progress, consult your physician to find out if there is a medical reason that is restricting your flexibility.

· The stretching exercises should each be done at least five times. Always blow all your breath out forcefully at the same time you bend and try to touch the floor in all of these exercises.

This maneuver moves the diaphragm up into the chest leaving less in the abdominal cavity to interfere with bending while reaching for the floor. Inhale as you resume the upright position.

Proceed through the remaining exercises without stopping. Adjust the rate of the exercises to avoid chest discomfort, excessive shortness of breath or exhaustion.

THE STRETCHING AND FLEXING EXERCISES

Exercise 9
This is a traditional exercise often used to demonstrate flexibility.

Stand with the feet slightly further apart than the width of the shoulders. Inhale, lift the arms and arch the back so as to see a spot on the ceiling behind you and feel the belly muscles stretching. At the peak of inhaling, begin blowing your breath out forcefully and bend the body forward in a continuous movement, without bending your knees. Try to touch the floor with the *palms* of the hands. (First try tips of fingers.) This will be difficult at first, but try at least five times at each session. Even if at first this does not seem possible, before long this will be easy for those who persevere.

Repeat this exercise at least five times.

Exercise 9

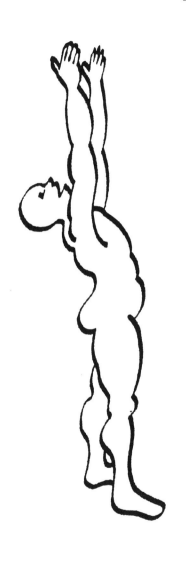

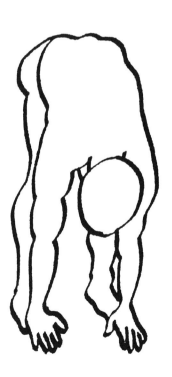

THE STRETCHING AND FLEXING EXERCISES

Exercise 10
This exercise introduces a slight twisting action while flexing the spine to help maintain a full range of motion.

Hold the left thumb in the right hand and stand with the feet slightly further apart than the width of the shoulders. Inhale, lift the arms and arch the back to see a spot on the ceiling behind you and feel the belly muscles stretching. This time while blowing your breath out forcefully and noisily, swing the extended arms and try to touch the right foot with the knuckles. Repeat trying to touch the left foot.

Repeat this exercise at least five times.

Exercise 10

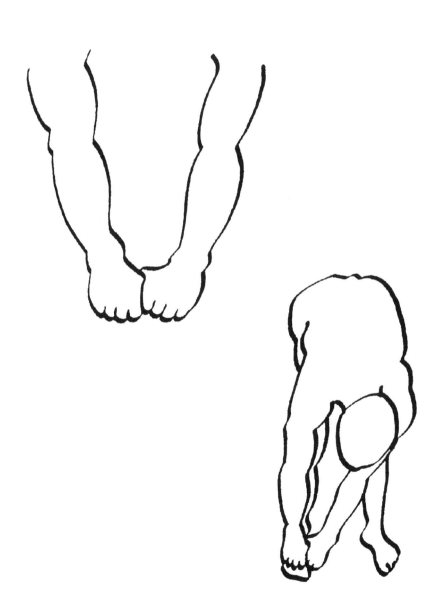

THE STRETCHING AND FLEXING EXERCISES

Exercise 11
This exercise continues as above and involves particularly the muscles of the buttocks and those in the front part of the neck.

Arch the back, swing the arms in an arc around to the back and place one hand on each buttocks. While still inhaling, tighten the muscles in the front of the neck and buttocks at the same time. It is surprising how the two sets of muscles can work together! Now exhale forcefully and swing the arms around to the front, bend forward and try to touch the floor with your knuckles.

Repeat this exercise at least five times.

Exercise 11

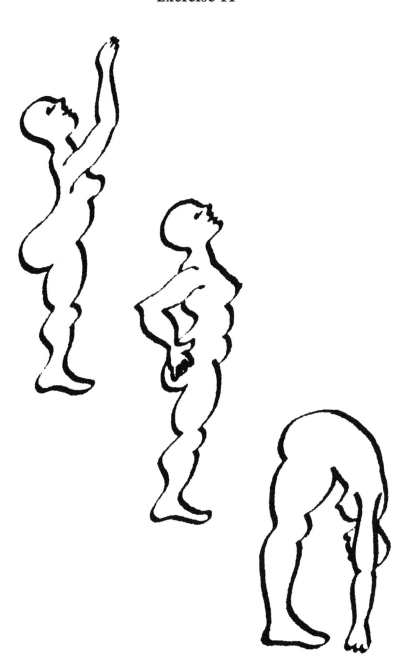

THE STRETCHING AND FLEXING EXERCISES

Exercise 12
This exercise again introduces a slight variation to involve additional muscles to further increase the range of motion.

Arch the back and lift the arms while inhaling but this time try to whistle as you exhale, bend forward and slide the left hand along the outside of the right leg until it reaches the ankle. Repeat the same with the right hand sliding the outside of the left leg.

Repeat this exercise at least five times.

Exercise 12

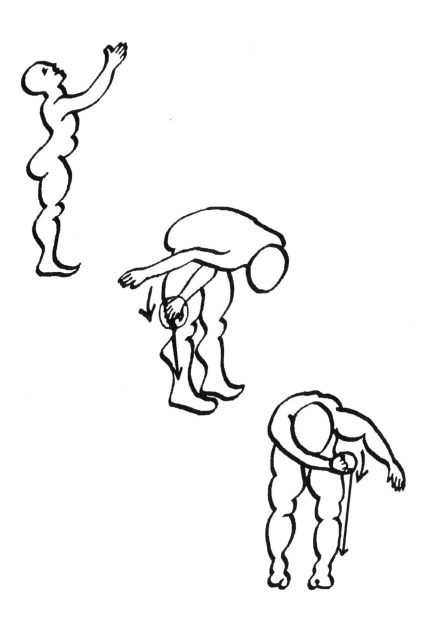

THE STRETCHING AND FLEXING EXERCISES

Exercise 13
This exercise introduces a twisting action involving the upper spine.

With arms extended to the sides, inhale, clench the fists and rotate the upper body to the left and rise to your toes. Now exhale, drop to your heels and relax your fists. Now repeat, but this time rotate to the right.

Repeat this exercise at least five times in each direction.

Exercise 13

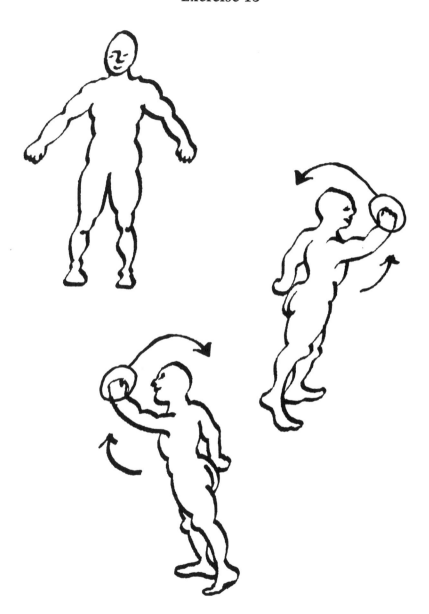

THE STRETCHING AND FLEXING EXERCISES

Exercise 14
This and the next exercise help maintain freely moving shoulder joints and stress the importance of coordinating respiration with muscle movements.

Extend your arms to the side, clench your fists and make four or five small clockwise circles with your arms. With each circle rise to your toes then drop your heels. Repeat this procedure with counter-clockwise circles. Repeat this combination four times. Now enlarge each circle to the maximum, ending in a counter-clockwise direction with hands in front.

Immediately proceed to the next exercise.

Note: It is important to breathe in with each series of clockwise arm rotations and breathe out with the counter clockwise rotations. With practice each series of rotations can be performed on a single slow inhalation and equally slow expiration. The entire series ends with arms and hands extended in front. At this point you have blown most of the air out of your lungs and must start to breathe in as you proceed to the next exercise.

Exercise 14

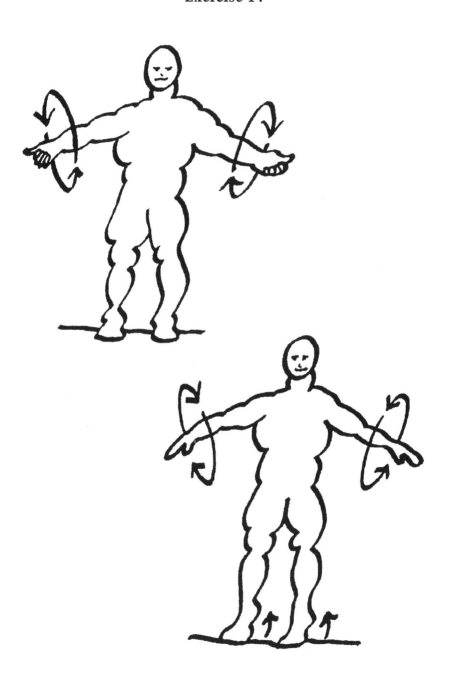

THE STRETCHING AND FLEXING EXERCISES

Exercise 15
This exercise aims to maintain flexibility of the upper body.

While breathing in bring the hands quickly over the head. At the same time arch the back. You will feel the belly muscles stretching as the momentum of the arm movement pulls you to your toes. Then bring your hands back down to the front and swing the arms rapidly to the sides while forcefully exhaling. You will feel the stretching of the muscles and ligaments around the shoulder joints. Now bring the hands back to the front.

Repeat this exercise at least five times.

Exercise 15

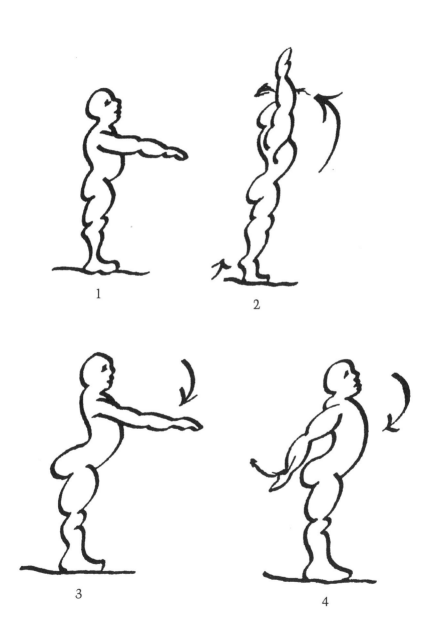

1

2

3

4

THE STRETCHING AND FLEXING EXERCISES

Exercise 16

Inhale, rise onto the toes and reach for the ceiling with the left clenched fist. Now exhale, relax the hand and drop from your toes as your arm falls to your side. Repeat reaching for the ceiling with the right fist.

Repeat this exercise at least five times with each arm.

Exercise 16

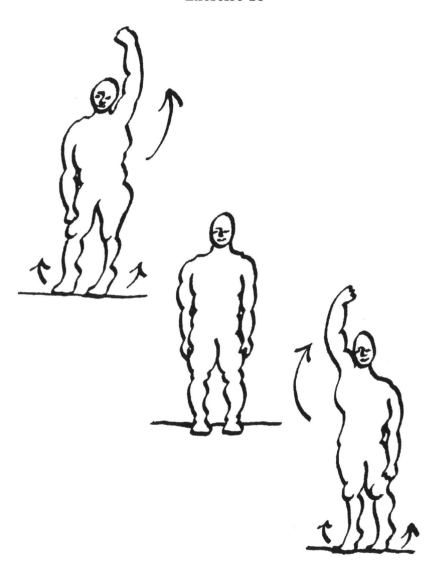

THE STRETCHING AND FLEXING EXERCISES

Exercise 17

Clasp the hands behind the back and raise them as high as possible. Inhale and rise onto the toes. Exhale, lower your hands, and drop from the toes.

Repeat this exercise at least five times.

Exercise 17

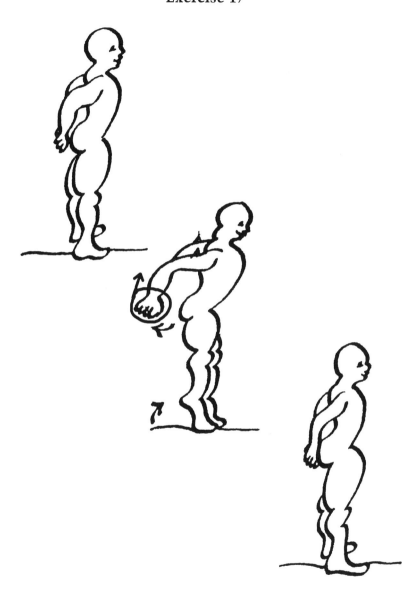

THE STRETCHING AND FLEXING EXERCISES

Exercise 18
This exercise involves muscles that are used to stand on the heels.

Try rocking from the toes to the heels. Use the arms to aid in maintaining balance. Inhale while rocking onto the heels and raising the arms. Now exhale as you drop the arms and rise onto the toes. If this exercise poses a problem in maintaining balance, place the hands on a wall for support during the exercise.

Repeat this exercise at least five times.

Exercise 18

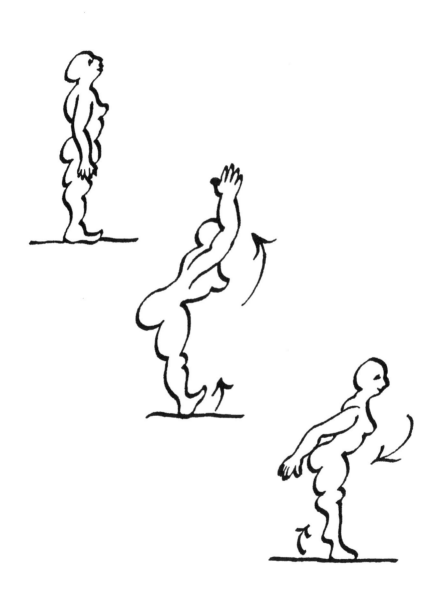

CHAPTER 6

The Isorobic Exercises

The stretching exercises are finished and we proceed to the unique *isorobic* exercises. These exercises replace weight lifting or resistance machines. Isorobic exercises increase the size and strength of the muscles. We attempt to use as many muscles of the body as possible with each exercise. This augments the beneficial effect of each exercise on the circulation.

It is especially important to correlate each *muscle contraction* with *inhalations* for reasons already discussed.

The number of times each of the following exercises are performed should be gradually increased until each is performed 20 times.

Contract the buttocks and rise to your toes with each isorobic exercise. This uses the big muscles of the lower extremities to augment the effect of the isorobic contractions of the upper extremity muscles in "squeezing" the blood out of the muscles into the veins leading to the heart.

The importance of coordination of inhalation with

muscle contraction is stressed again. The inhalation is not as deep as in the stretching exercises, but must be simultaneous with each muscle contraction.

Adjust the depth and rate of inspiration to prevent overbreathing which can cause a feeling of faintness or giddiness. If this occurs, stop momentarily and resume the exercises at a slower pace. The intensity and the number of times each exercise is performed depends on the state of general health and fitness when the program is started.

The duration of each muscle contraction and inspiration is equal.

Avoid excessive shortness of breath, pain or tightness in the chest or pain in any joint. If properly done and properly coordinated with respiration as directed, these exercises will provide benefits similar to those of most aerobic muscle toning exercises. There is no need for special apparatus.

There is less increase in work for the heart with significant increase in blood flow to the vital organs. The entire exercise program is not exhausting and therefore, more acceptable to most people.

Gradually increase each exercise to a minimum of 20 times.

THE ISOROBIC EXERCISES

Exercise 19

Start with palms facing the ceiling, forearms parallel to the floor and elbows held close to the body. Inhale, rise to the toes, contract the buttocks, clench the fists and attempt to further flex the forearms against an imaginary resistance that prevents further flexing. Feel and see the forearm muscles tighten and at the same time the muscles in the front and back of the upper arm tighten. All these muscles should contract simultaneously. Very little further flexing of the forearms will occur. Now exhale, settle back from your toes and relax the muscles but keep the forearms flexed at 90 degrees.

Repeat the entire process up to 20 times.

Be sure to get up on your toes and contract the buttocks with each muscle contraction.

Repeat 20 times.

Exercise 19

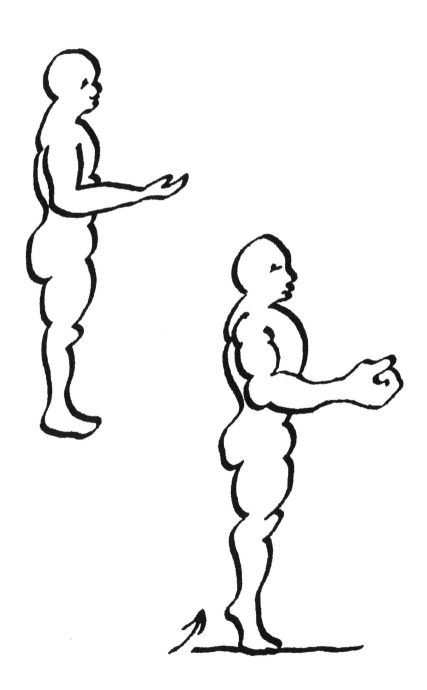

THE ISOROBIC EXERCISES

Exercise 20

Hold arms with forearms flexed as in previous exercise, but this time hold the elbows slightly toward the front and away from the body. Inhale, contract the buttocks, rise onto the toes and try to bring the elbows together against an imaginary resistance. Feel the muscles in the shoulders, upper back and chest contract as they resist bringing the elbows to the side of the body. Now exhale, relax.

Repeat the entire process up to 20 times.

Exercise 20

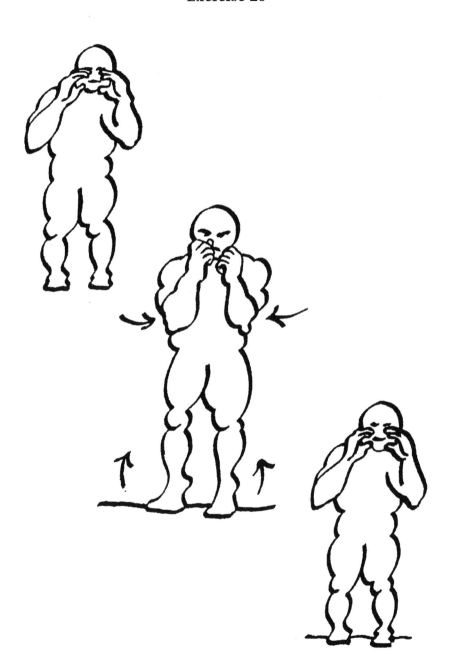

THE ISOROBIC EXERCISES

Exercise 21

Hold arms out front at shoulder level with elbows bent, forearms flexed and fingers of hands interlocked. Pull one hand against the other, contract the buttocks, rise onto the toes and inhale. Drop from your toes; relax your hands and arms as you exhale.

Repeat 20 times.

Exercise 21

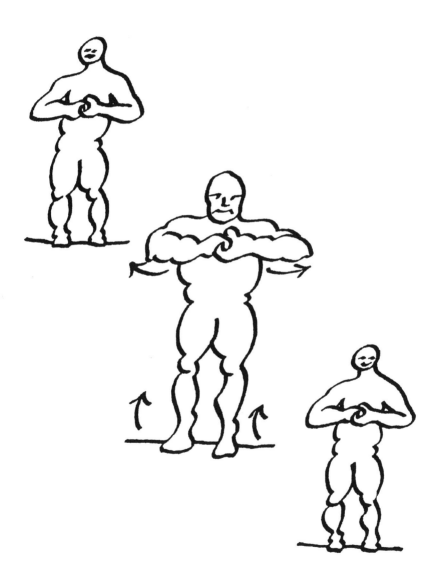

THE ISOROBIC EXERCISES

Exercise 22

Hold arms out front at shoulder level with elbows bent. Clasp hands and push one against the other as you inhale, contract buttocks and rise onto the toes. Relax, exhale, and drop from your toes.

Repeat 20 times.

Exercise 22

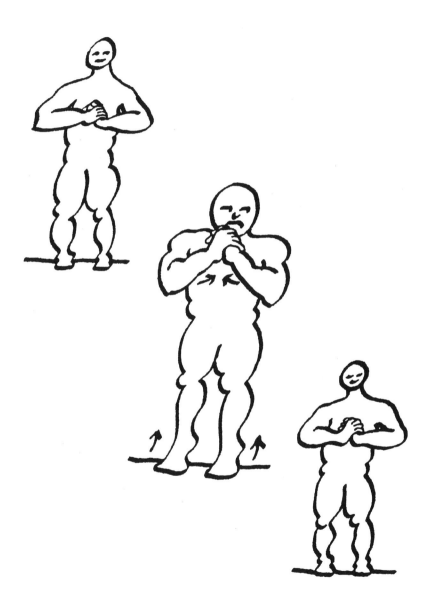

THE ISOROBIC EXERCISES

Exercise 23

With left forearm flexed at right angle, hold left elbow against the side of the body. Place the right palm on top of the left palm and push downward as the left hand is trying to push up. The position of the left elbow does not change during this maneuver which is performed as you inhale, contract buttocks and rise to your toes. Now relax the pressure, drop from the toes and exhale.

Repeat 20 times.

Exercise 23

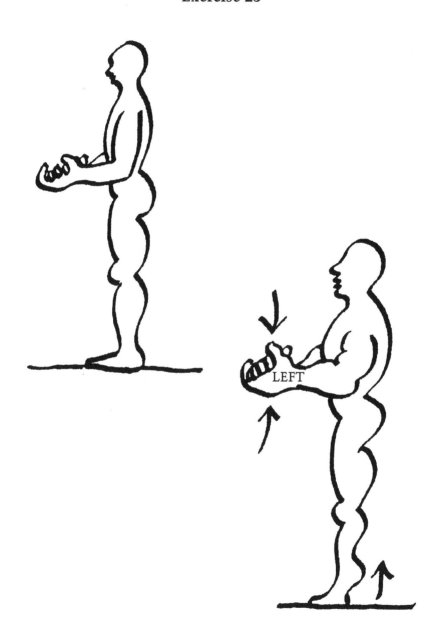

THE ISOROBIC EXERCISES

Exercise 24

With right forearm flexed at right angle, right elbow held against the side of the body, place the left palm on top of the right palm and push downward as the right hand is trying to push up. The position of the right elbow does not change during this maneuver which is performed as you inhale, contract buttocks and rise to your toes. Now relax the pressure, drop from the toes and exhale.

Repeat 20 times.

Exercise 24

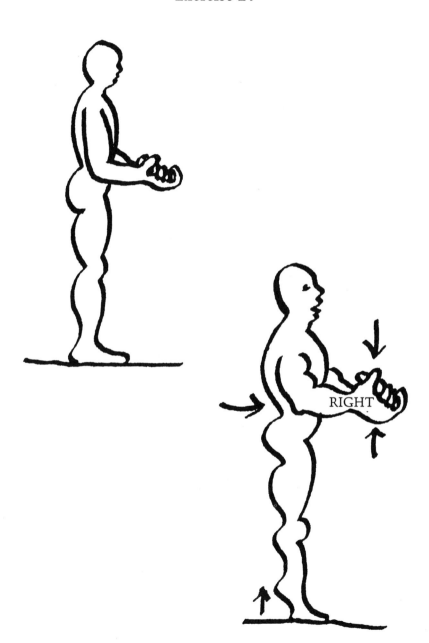

THE ISOROBIC EXERCISES

Exercise 25

Hold the arms out in front, elbows pointing outward, forearms at approximately right angels to the upper arms and fists closed. Now contract the muscles between the shoulder blades and resist having the shoulders and elbows pulled backward. At the same time rise onto the toes, contract buttocks and inhale. Feel the contraction of the muscles between the shoulder blades and a pull in front of the shoulders as the pectoral muscles contract to keep the arms from being pulled backward. Now drop from the toes, exhale and relax the muscles.

Repeat 20 times.

Exercise 25

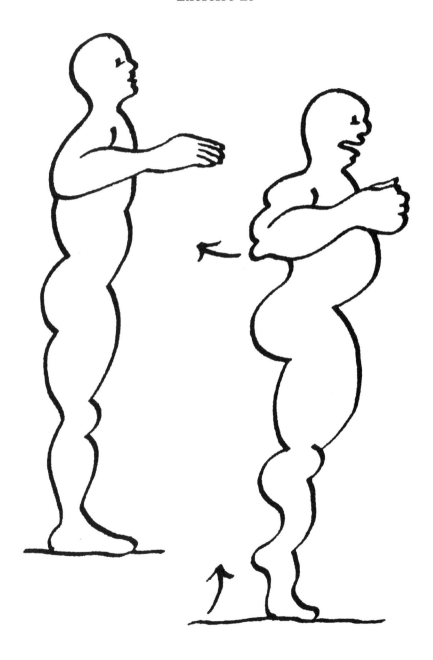

THE ISOROBIC EXERCISES

Exercise 26

Hold the arms out in front, elbows pointing outward, forearms at approximately right angles to
the upper arms and fists closed, concentrate on
contracting the muscles on the back of the upper
arms (the triceps) and the muscles in back of the
neck. Resist straightening the arms as all the
muscles in the arms and neck are contracting and
you rise onto your toes and contract the buttocks.
You should feel the contraction of the neck
muscles extending to the base of the skull. Exhale as muscles are relaxed and the body is low-
ered to the floor.

Repeat 20 times.

Exercise 26

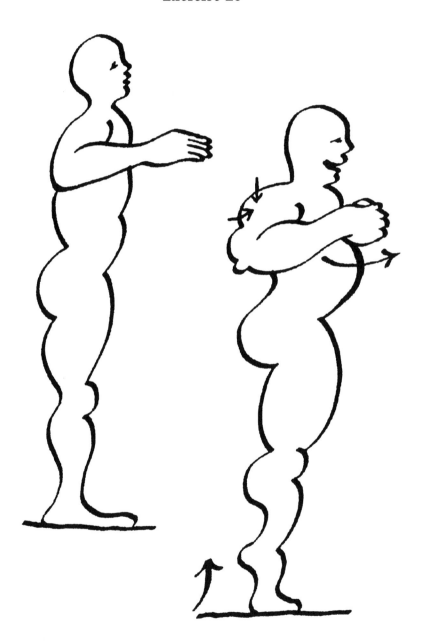

THE ISOROBIC EXERCISES

Exercise 27
This exercise aims to improve balance and strengthen the lower extremity muscles.

Squatting exercises maintain the flexibility of the lower extremity joints and strengthen the lower extremity muscles. Place the arms at the sides of the body, make a fist, rise to the toes and inhale. Now extend the arms in front parallel to the floor, open the fists, squat with back straight and exhale. Use the extended arms as a balancing aid and fix the eyes on some object while squatting down. If balance remains a problem, hold on to a chair during this exercise. Now inhale, bring the arms to the sides with closed fist and rise to erect position.

Gradually increase the number of squats to 10.

Exercise 27

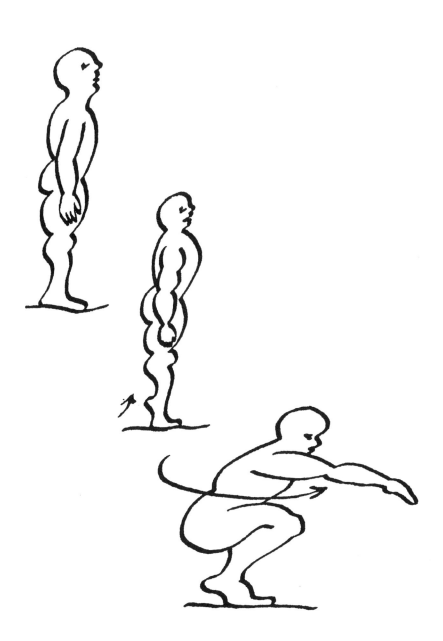

THE ISOROBIC EXERCISES

Exercise 28
This exercise increases the flexibility of the knee joints and aids balance.

Try to bring the knee up, grasp the ankle and pull it up and push the thigh toward the body. Alternate knees. Blow out the breath as the knee is pulled toward the chest. This will require balancing on one foot as the other foot is raised and the ankle and leg are pulled toward the chest. <u>Do not attempt this exercise if balance is a problem.</u>

Repeat 20 times.

Exercise 28

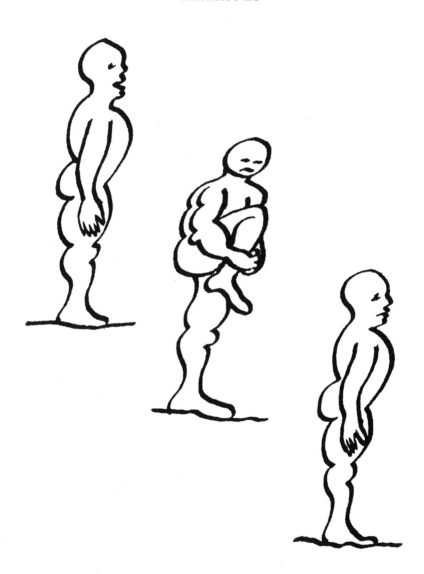

THE ISOROBIC EXERCISES

Exercise 29

The traditional "push up" will further improve the tone and strength of the upper body muscles. *Breathe in* during the push up and exhale as the body moves toward the floor. It may be advisable for some to start with the "half push-up" by keeping the knees on the floor and pushing up only the upper half of the body. The number of push-ups should be increased as tolerated.

Repeat 20 times.

The entire exercise program should be carried out without a stop. There is no magic to the order in which the isorobic exercises are done, but it is advisable to do them in the same sequence each time. This will help in making the entire routine almost automatic. The number of times each exercise is performed should produce moderate shortness of breath. This may require increasing the number and intensity of each exercise with time. There is little to be gained by extending the duration of exercising beyond 30 minutes, except to risk boredom! It is more productive to augment the program by other activities.

This program will maintain flexibility of joints, improve muscle tone and strength and produce a sense of well being. With the addition of a brisk walk, a round of golf or a game of doubles tennis two or three times a week, a remarkable degree of fitness can be attained without exhaustion and with little risk. All this is a bonus. The primary purpose of the program is to increase the flow of fresh, oxygen-rich blood to the heart and brain.

CHAPTER 7

Other Factors
Affecting
Your Health

The primary aim of the program outlined in the first six chapters is to improve the circulation to the heart muscle and the brain.

The physical fitness resulting from the program is a bonus. In the last analysis the success of any attempt to increase blood flow through the coronary arteries depends to a major degree on healthy, wide open arteries.

It has been scientifically established that a high saturated fat, high cholesterol diet plays a major role in premature obstruction of coronary and other important arteries. An appropriate diet should, therefore, accompany this exercise program. It is not the purpose of this book to provide details of an ideal diet. Many books have been written on ideal diets. However, they do not all agree on what constitutes an ideal diet. Some general comments about factors that may influence compliance with a general good health program may prove to be helpful.

A practical guide in this field is to imagine the human

body as a very complicated, sophisticated chemical plant, as it deals with nutrition.

As managers of this chemical plant, it is our responsibility to provide the appropriate raw material. A healthy "plant" can, within reason, select what is required for the good nutritional health of the body and excrete what it does not need. One must not overwhelm the plant with excessive loads of unnecessary and undesirable raw material and yet be certain that the essential elements are supplied.

To this end, a diet low in saturated fats, high in fiber, fruit and vegetables is generally recommended to meet these requirements. The following suggestions are reasonable adjuncts to such a diet.

(1) Avoid large meals of any composition, even low fat. Large meals distend the stomach and intestines and make it more difficult to breathe. Heavy meals require more blood for the digestive process and may steal blood essential for vital organs including the heart and brain. This may result in unhappy consequences for anyone with borderline blood supply to the brain and heart.

(2) When eating at restaurants and unable to resist the "clean plate ethic," divide the entree in half and make up your mind that one half will go into a doggy bag before the first bite is taken. Most restaurants serve much larger portions than most people eat at home.

(3) Older digestive systems handle "rich foods" poorly. Rich foods are the ones that make you feel uncomfortably full and bloated. They are also the foods which generally contain more fat than you should eat. Why eat foods which

make you feel uncomfortable and are very likely to elevate the blood cholesterol level?

(4) Avoid the obvious cholesterol traps, such as eggs, fat rich dairy products and organ meats. This does not mean always!

(5) Drink only skim milk, which contains all the nutritional value of whole milk without the undesirable fat. It takes a short time to become accustomed to skim milk.

(6) Poultry with skin removed provides the protein and other nutrients with much less fat than other meats. Fish is always a desirable protein source because it does not contain saturated fats that the body converts to cholesterol. If you count calories, the total fat calories should aim at approximately 20 percent total daily caloric intake. Diets with as little as 10 percent of the calories in fat can reduce the cholesterol blood level and actually improve the state of the coronary and other arteries. Such extreme fat restriction is difficult to maintain and may not be safe. Similar results may be obtained with a more reasonable diet and the use of drugs if diet alone fails to control cholesterol levels.

(7) Try different breakfast foods, such as fish, tuna salad or chicken on a toasted English muffin or water bagel. The traditional American breakfast of bacon or ham and eggs should be relegated to special occasions.

(8) Eat fresh fruits for snacks and desserts. Even a carrot can satisfy that between meal desire to eat "something," which is often really a desire to "*do*" something.

(9) The role of alcohol in health and disease has recently received a great deal of attention in lay and medical literature. What has not been stressed is that alcohol contains more calories per gram than the starches. Calorie counters may not realize that in the "two martini lunch," a good part of the allotted lunch calories has been consumed before the first bite has been taken. Perhaps Samuel Johnson had it right when about 200 years ago he allegedly said, "All the virtue of alcohol resides in the first ounce or two," but he was not talking about calories. Johnson has many supporters who maintain that a drink or two per day may be good for the heart.

(10) A word in defense of salt intake may be helpful. First, salt (sodium chloride) is essential to the body chemistry. Complete elimination of salt from the diet, if possible, would be disastrous. Most people can handle a reasonable intake of salt without risk. Indeed under certain conditions it is essential to replace salt lost by excessive perspiration.

On the other hand there are some people with certain diseases, which are characterized by the body's inability to adjust the body levels of sodium. In these situations even modest amounts of salt presented to the body cannot be handled appropriately and the blood sodium may rise above normal levels. This generally results in fluid retention and swelling which may be generalized or restricted to the lower extremities. Obviously these people should restrict salt intake and seek professional advice.

(11) Recent medical studies have suggested that some vitamins and minerals known as antioxidants may delay the onset or progression of degenerative vascular conditions.

Since there is no evidence that these vitamins and minerals in the recommended doses are harmful, it appears safe to go on the following vitamin regime. Take one capsule of multivitamin with minerals per day along with 400 units of vitamin E, 500 mgs. of vitamin C and 50 mgs. of Zinc. Many other supplements such as Selenium and herbal products are being recommended. Some recommendations have very little scientific justification. Not all have been proven to be safe. If taking those products that are proven to be safe do not put too great a strain on the pocketbook or upset the stomach, it will do no harm and may possibly be proven in the future to do some good.

(12) Obesity is a negative for general health and more specifically for coronary heart disease. The American public spends almost as much money in trying to find an easy way to lose weight as it does on trying to find an easy way to stay fit. In many instances these efforts join paths. Although exercise should be an important component in any weight loss program, it is not the secret to weight loss success. A person who weighs more than 20 percent above the norm for that person's sex, age, and body skeletal build is considered obese. Every extra pound of body fat requires the heart to provide not only the extra blood to the muscles that carry the additional weight, but also blood to keep the fat cells alive. In this respect a person who is 40 pounds overweight is putting a greater burden on the heart than a person who is forced to constantly carry a 40 pound weight which requires no blood to keep it alive. It is obvious that people with heart disease should make every effort to maintain normal or slightly below normal body weight. This is often no easy task for the obese person. The causes of obesity are many and complicated. Much remains to be learned

about obesity and weight loss. One thing is certain: there are no magic crash diets that will cure obesity. Heart disease is often a potent motivator. Patients who strive unsuccessfully to control their weight suddenly find they are able to do so after a heart attack. In the current state of our knowledge or ignorance, the best course of action for the obese person who must lose weight is to avoid crash diets and consult a dietician recommended by a physician.

AND SO, DO THE "HEART FRIENDLY EXERCISES." EAT WISELY. YOU WILL LIVE LONGER, FEEL YOUNGER AND BE HAPPIER!

About the Author

Dr. Jack Wexler graduated from The Medical College of Virginia. He completed his postgraduate training with a research fellowship in cardiovascular diseases on the Harvard Services of the Boston City Hospital. During the Second World War he served as Chief of Cardiovascular Service at Ft. Devons Station Hospital in Massachusetts. He later served as Chief of the Medical Section and Executive Officer of the Chemical Warfare Service at Edgewood Arsenal in Maryland.

Post war he was a physician at the Johns Hopkins Hospital and a part-time faculty member of the Johns Hopkins Medical School. He was a consultant in cardiology to the Veterans Hospital at Ft. Howard, Maryland.

Dr. Wexler is board certified in both Cardiology and Internal Medicine. For over thirty years he was in the private practice of cardiology in Baltimore, Maryland.

He has received several honors including: Election to Phi Beta Kappa and Alpha Epsilon Delta, an honorary medical school society. He was the recipient of a Cardiology research grant from the National Institute of Health.

He has published a number of scientific articles in leading medical journals.

Dr. Wexler currently lives on Longboat Key, Florida,

with his wife of fifty-four years. They maintain both mental and physical fitness by their daily heart friendly exercises, golf, walks and being involved in local affairs.